Exercises for
Hearing Mindfully
Volume Two

Mindfulness Practices for Persons
with Parkinson's Disease

9/3/2014
Parkinsons Recovery
Robert Rodgers PhD

Contents

© Parkinsons Recovery

The Parkinsons Recovery Mindfulness Series

Realistically speaking, how can the intense level of stress that aggravates the symptoms of Parkinson's disease be calmed? Better yet, how can they be quieted? My research over the past decade reveals that using your mind to drop the stress level down a notch or two always backfires. When you tell yourself:

- *Settle down!*
- *Take it easy!*
- *Stop being so stressed out!*

The stress level ratchets up, not down. Attempts to force the stress and anxiety levels to adjust downward induce an internally generated stress. They pile more stress on top of an excess of stress that already exists. There are certainly a sufficient number of external generators of stress in every one's life. Why infuse more stress that you create yourself, even with the best of intentions?

If the mind is not a useful technique to reduce stress, what is? The most eloquent answer I have for you is to become more mindful of what is experienced in the present moment. Becoming more mindful shifts you into the experience of the "now" which in itself is less stressful (unless you have been kidnapped by terrorists!).

It is stressful to anticipate events you imagine will occur in the future. The events we imagine rarely happen. Does this ring true for you? We all create unnecessary stress in our lives by how and where we focus our thoughts and attention.

It is stressful to agonize over the past. When we think about the past, we are much more likely to think about unpleasant experiences that induce stress. The past event itself was traumatic enough. Yet, we insist on reliving the trauma over and over again through our memories. It seems some of us just can't get enough stress in our lives.

The problem with upping the ante on stress levels is that – as you well know – symptoms of Parkinson's disease become worse. When you are not as stressed, your symptoms are far less problematic.

I have reached one solid conclusion from my ten years of research on Parkinson's disease. Symptoms will drive you crazy when you are stressed and are far less problematic when stress is under control.

Now, if you can't use your mind to become more mindful (which creates added stress in itself) how in the world can you quiet down a frantic lifestyle? I have concluded that the simplest and most effective solution to reducing stress levels is to become more mindful.

Exercises for Hearing Mindfully
Mindfulness Practices for Persons with Parkinson's Disease
Volume Two

The transformation is possible step by step through these simple exercises you can do anywhere, anytime of the day. The Parkinsons Recovery mindfulness exercises are designed to focus your attention on the present moment as attention on either the past or the future is diverted. A renewed focus on the present moment reduces stress levels. Mindfulness is a lifestyle that will reduce stresses in your life if you set the intention to take a mindfulness practice seriously.

I recommend that you practice each of the exercises for a week or longer. Incorporate each practice into your regular routines and habits. Attempts to do all of the exercises simultaneously will likely induce more stress which – obviously – is contrary to the intent of a successful mindfulness program.

Give each exercise a little time and space. Invite the stresses in your life to dissipate. Allow the experience of each practice to engulf you. In so doing, watch the stresses in your life dip down to new lows along with a concurrent relief of any and all symptoms that you have currently been experiencing.

This volume is one out of nine I have developed to support the recovery of persons who currently experience neurological symptoms. A full listing of the Parkinsons Recovery Mindfulness booklets follows:

4

Exercises for Hearing Mindfully
Mindfulness Practices for Persons with Parkinson's Disease
Volume Two

Robert Rodgers, PhD

Parkinsons Recovery

www.parkinsonsrecovery.me

Olympia, Washington

Mindful Listening

The mindfulness challenge that I have for you this week is to become a sponge when listening to friends, family and co-workers as they talk. Listen with your entire body, your heart and your essence. Listen as if you were a sponge.

1. **Hear every nuance.**
2. **See every gesture.**
3. **Notice every pause.**
4. **Sense every emotion.**
5. **Soak up every word.**

No responses need be offered or given, even if solicited.

When another person talks "at us", it is not uncommon to extend to them a tiny fraction of our full attention. We half-way listen to what they are saying as we ponder the many unfinished tasks that remain to be done by the end of the day. We are all guilty!

How many conversations do you typically have with other people that are unsatisfying? How often do you feel as though you have not been heard? How frequently do you realize that the person is only partially attentive to what it is you are trying to communicate? How often does the other person claim that they understand you, but you know in your heart that they do not come close?

© Parkinsons Recovery

When you do communicate with others this week - be a sponge. Notice any thoughts that float into your mind as you listen. Simply acknowledge each and every thought as it emerges whatever it might be. Place each thought in a "holding" container as you continue listening.

As a person talks you might notice they have -

- *Wrinkles or*
- *A scratchy face or*
- *Moles under their left ear*

Perhaps you think to yourself -

> *"My goodness. My friend is looking much older today than they did the last time I saw them last month."*

Thoughts do pop into our heads that have nothing to do with what the person is attempting to communicate. There is no practical way to stop those thoughts. When they do slip into your head, simply say to yourself -

> *"Oh, right. Okay, let me just put this thought aside and re-direct my attention to absorbing all that this person is saying that I'm talking with right now. I want to hear all the words. I want to understand their true intent. I want to get the full meaning."*

To become a sponge means to -

1. *Absorb all the words*
2. *Be fully and completely present*
3. *Hear every idea the person is trying to convey*
4. *Understand the true meaning of their words*
5. *Honor the feelings underneath their words*

It may well be the case that there are situations where you do have to make decisions. Of course you need to do that. But, in other instances when you are communicating with another individual, be a sponge. Get the full experience of what it means to devote your full energy, attention and essence to what the other person is attempting to say. Not everyone is a word smith. Sometimes you have to listen with your heart.

Deeper Meaning Behind Mindful Listening

How has the mindfulness challenge this week to listen like a sponge been going? I'm guessing that your comfort level with this mindfulness challenge will be a function of your background and education. If you are a lawyer or a judge, this assignment and challenge would have been particularly challenging. You have been trained to always respond, argue, debate and criticize. This is also true of academics, the foundation of my own background and experience. If you are a therapist, artist or musician the challenge might not have been quite so difficult.

8

Therapists are trained and experienced at fully and completely devoting their full attention to another person. Artists and musicians are trained to go with the flow so to speak.

Have you avoided the challenge? Did you forget about it? Have you engaged it? If so, what has been your experience?

I am hoping that there has been at least one encounter that you have had over the last several days when the other person sucked your energy with a war of words that allowed no opportunity for you to even respond or reply even if you wanted. In such circumstances, the urgent need is to make up an excuse to get away from the person. My response is typically -

"I have a meeting. Sorry. Have to go now."

Of course – the meeting is often with myself, but I am familiar company and we get much done, the two of us.

There are people in my life just like the person I described above. I suspect there are people in your life as well. There are people who are experts at sucking the energy of other people. There is no exchange of energy. With each and every encounter, it feels as though such persons have sharp claws that grab into our physical body and pull out any and all remnants of energy that remain within.

9

Individuals who make it a practice to suck the life force of others have what is described as an oral personality; they have been abandoned at one point or another in their life. We need to have forgiveness and compassion for such individuals. Many people carry the wound of abandonment.

Still, it is very challenging to be around such persons for longer than a few minutes. I can personally be depleted of all my energy in a matter of five minutes. My energy depletes and drains quickly. Has this possibly happened with you? Have you thought to yourself -

> *"Oh, my God, I can't be a sponge any longer; I've got to exit this particular conversation."*

Or, did you have to abort the mindfulness challenge altogether? Did you find an excuse to leave? Did you just stop listening like a sponge? Did you get angry? Or, did you somehow interact in a way that allowed for the encounter to be suspended or terminated?

Why am I hoping that this particular experience might have been one that you have had over the last several days? It is actually similar to our reactions when we have no choice but to listen to our own body communicate messages of distress and pain.

Perhaps it is the case that your body is sending out many signals today of pain and discomfort. Perhaps you are feeling, frankly speaking, lousy. What are you going to do in response to this lousy day? Are you going to want to try to get away from the messages your body is trying to communicate? Most people do. Do you think about taking a vacation so that you don't have to be living with your body? Many of us have had those feelings when we feel lousy.

We can always get away from another person using one excuse or another or just walk away. It is, unfortunately, never possible to take a vacation from our body. Many people check-out in the sense that they stop listening to their bodies. They say to themselves,

> *"Boy, things are really haywire in there. I'm really angry at you. I'm going to go to somewhere and get this fixed."*

There is then a frantic rush to find somebody out there who can work some magic to relieve the symptoms that are being experienced. No quick fix exists for most people, so this response usually leads to more frustration.

The real challenge for the rest of the week is to be fully and completely present to all of the messages your body is communicating to you, moment to moment. Be fully and completely present to all messages and information that your body is sending in the form of symptoms.

Perhaps there is a tremor in your right hand. Connect with that tremor. Ask your hand, just as if it were a person,

> *"What's up? Talk to me, let me know what's going on."*

Ask your body (as if it were another person) to give you the information you need to understand what in the world might be causing the tremoring. You can do this with any symptom whether it is -

1. *Pain due to stiffness*
2. *Difficulty with walking*
3. *Challenges with swallowing*
4. *Embarrassment due to tremors*

It does not matter what the symptom is. Connect with the organ, limb or muscle in your body that is problematic in the moment. Instead of running away from the challenge -

Connect with it.

Become a sponge.

Ask your body to say more.

> *"Hello? Help me out. What's going on here?"*

12

Engage in an authentic dialogue. Some therapies treat symptoms by masking them. The cause remains undiscovered and untreated. Over time symptoms will worsen.

The challenge for recovery is to go a step further and to ask,

> *"What is causing this symptom? What's really going on here? What do I need to change about my life to be able to correct the problem that is causing the symptoms that I am currently experiencing?"*

There is no simple solution. There are no simple answers. The factors that create the symptoms of Parkinson's are multi-faceted. They are indeed complicated and convoluted.

It is possible and doable to chip away at the causes little by little. How do we do that? We become a sponge. We treat our body as if our body were another person. We connect fully and completely with the full essence of what our body is trying to communicate to us. This is how we figure out what is causing the symptoms. This is also how we figure out what to do about it.

Our body is a miracle. Our body knows how to heal. When the body is out of balance, it is not its normal state. Wellness and balance is.

Become a sponge.

1. *1.*   *Connect*
2. *2.*   *Listen*
3. *3.*   *Receive*

Your body is giving you information every minute of your life. Listen to your body as if you were a sponge, just as you have been listening to others communicate their concerns to you this week. Extend to your body the precious opportunity to heal. You will be amazed and dazzled at the result.

Mindful Attention to Distractors

My challenge for you this week promises to be totally and completely fun and, at the same time, totally and completely frustrating. My invitation is for you to begin hearing and acknowledging all of the qualifiers that you use when you talk. Hear qualifiers when you speak like "uh" and "so" for example.

The most common utterance used in the English language is "uh." When you say "uh" or when you say, "so..." or when you say "what I mean is..." you are creating distractions from what it is that you truly intend for the listener to hear. You are distracting yourself from your true intent and you are distracting your listeners.

When I began the Parkinsons Recovery radio program, it took some months to become familiar with how my voice sounded to me when I edited the recordings. What I heard was not what I was accustomed to hearing when I talk. The true surprise as it turns out was the many, many qualifiers that I use when I talk. Quite frankly, I was shocked.

I began counting the number of "uhh...uhh...uhs" that I used when I talked and I was flabbergasted. What I'd like to invite you to do is to begin noticing as you talk how many qualifiers you use when you speak.

A second invitation which has the promise to be quite fun is to engage a family member or friend in this particular challenge. Ask them for a day, an evening or an afternoon to catch each and every qualifier that you use. Of course, you could ask them to be very specific and to alert you as to when you use a very specific qualifier like "uh," or you could simply ask them to raise a finger every time you use any particular phrase that they believe is a distractor.

Or, instead of alerting you each time you could ask a family member or friend to make a secret count. For example, as you begin dinnertime they could see how many qualifiers you have used which they tally up by the end of the meal.

Please don't be overwhelmed by this assignment. If this is all you are mindful about, it could potentially drive you nuts.

Another possibility you may want to consider is to record yourself when you actually talk, even in casual conversations, and then listen to the recording afterward. It is likely you will discover just as I did that you do use many qualifiers when you talk.

This week, then, become mindful of all of those distracting words -- those unnecessary words -- that add nothing to your true intent. Notice those distractions when you converse with another person. Include in this challenge certain profanity words that really do not add to the point that you are intending to make (unless of course they help to emphasize your meaning!).

Have fun and please do not be completely frustrated with this. I hope you find it to be a fun and exhilarating assignment which invites to become much more mindful of each and every word that you speak. Your thoughts are precious to others and to yourself. Treat them as such.

Deeper Meaning Behind Distractors

What is the underlying meaning of the assignment this week to be more attentive to all words and expressions of distraction? Words of distraction actually deflate the effectiveness of the intent that we wish to convey. How many times have you listened to a person talk who uses so many qualifiers that you held the thought,

> *"Can't you just get the point? I really can't wait another 5 minutes for you to be able to use the words that I need to hear to understand what it is that you are actually saying."*

When we use many qualifying utterances in the sentences that we speak to others, our thoughts are not taken seriously. People in the public arena such as television announcers practice talking so that they don't use qualifiers and distractors. They well know that their

17

audience will stop listening after a couple of sentences if their sentences are filled with words like "uh," and "well" and "what I mean is…"

There is another, much more important reason to become mindful of qualifiers that you inject when you talk. You are using these same qualifiers when you think about the possibility of recovery. I, as you know, interview hundreds of people every year about their thoughts with regard to recovery.

I often ask the question,

> "So how is fairing, how is recovery looking for you?"

The answers that I hear are clues about the real intent the person has set for recovery. For example, I'm going to now paraphrase some of what I have heard over the last decade:

> "Well, you know, the doctor says that it's really not going to be possible, so of course, you know, I'm going to him for a long time and I know, um, that well, he's you know, pretty prestigious guy, he's, you know, well, he's at a really, I mean, uh, a really good university and I, well you know, I--I really got the best man, and--and, that I could possibly get. And so, I don't know, I just hope that uh, well, I

> *don't know, I just hope that down the rod that uh, I*
> *guess if I could just not get--get worse, I mean, you*
> *know. You know that would be really--that's I'm*
> *like, well, like, I mean that's what really, that's*
> *what I guess in the end I'd like--I'd like to see."*

Maybe you think this is an exaggeration, but I assure you it is not. When people respond, there are qualifications that are embedded in how they express themselves. There are a string of distracting terms that take away from their true intention to recover. Contrast that response with the following, the question:

> *"How do you see the prospects for your recovery*
> *now?"*

Here's the answer:

> *"I'm recovering everyday – there's no doubt about*
> *it."*

End of story. That's it. That is all there is to the answer. That is the gist of the intention. No qualifying terms are needed or necessary. Contrast this response with:

> *"Well, yeah, you know, um, well, the way it turns*
> *out is I think all things considered, probably, you*
> *know, well, what people – what a lot of people*
> *really say is that they, they think I'm probably*

better, that I'm recovering and, you know, I don't know, I don't know exactly, well, I'd say, yeah, I'd probably, yeah, I'm recov--I do have, well, like everyone I have, you know, I have, I have bad-- some bad days here and there, but I guess I'm--I'm probably, yeah, I'm probably recovering. I--I guess, yep, I suppose that's right."

Now, I don't know how you felt about the contrast of those two responses but in just reading them it is profound for me. In the second response I am full of reservation and hesitation. I quite frankly do not have the true intent to take the action that is needed and required to be able to begin to reverse any symptoms whatever they may be.

In the very first statement there is absolutely no doubt but that in my heart, mind and soul and in every cell of my body I have set the intention to take whatever action is needed to reverse my symptoms and become symptom-free.

1. **I am ready to live my life.**
2. **I am ready to actualize my passion.**
3. **I am ready to activate my life force.**

There is a huge difference between the two statements. The first statement facilitates movement into that space of full power - that place where the intention for recovery is fully and completely activated.

It helps enormously to begin noticing all of the qualifiers that you use when you talk to anyone about anything. And, of course, as you begin to notice those qualifiers - as you talk out loud to others – those unconscious expressions of doubt and hesitation are the very same qualifiers that you are using when you talk to yourself about reversing your symptoms.

Let me know conclude with another contrast, a contrast with a statement that is full distractions and a final salutation that is not:

> *"So, uh, okay everybody out there. So, you know, well, this is Robert and well, I just it's been kind of-- it's, you know, everyone says it's been fun for me to do these and I know kind of like a--like everybody out there, you know, like, you know, you're listening and I, uh, so uh, you know I know that you probably uh, probably like this one, I don't know. And I really, I don't know whether you like, eh, shoot, I really I don't know whether you really liked it or not, but--but I did, you know, you know I thought it was, I--this was fun. Yeah, but there's no--yep, yeah, uh-huh, this was yep, no doubt about it. This was, this was just a whole lot of fun and anyway, so, uh this, uh, this is uh, Parkinsons*

Recovery and uh, I'm Robert and so, you know, like uh, have a really good week.

Now, let me see if I can contrast a very different salutation; a way that we can end our connection with one another today:

> *"I have fully and completely relished thinking about what I might assign to you as a challenge this week. I have been thrilled at the challenge I gave myself. I have found it fun and challenging. I know that you will also enjoy the experience. Have fun. Be challenged. Don't get too frustrated. Whatever you do, have a wonderful time.*

There is a big difference between the two for me as I speak and write these two statements. How about you?

Notice Sounds

Depending on our physiological make-up, our background and our genes, each of us has a preference for how we take in information from the world. Some of us are visual. I am raising my hands because that is my own preference. We take in information through our eyes, through sights and through images. Whenever we enter into a new space we see what is there primarily. Noises are secondary. Touch is tertiary.

Some of us however aren't seers or visual people. Their nature is to be auditory. They take in information through their ears. They process information through sound.

Finally, some people are kinesthetic which means that neither visual stimuli nor auditory stimuli tend to have much punch. The primary sensory input for kinesthetic people is through touch. When anybody, any person, any entity, any living creature is touched, a wealth of information is conveyed to the person who is kinesthetic.

The mindfulness challenge today and this week is primarily for individuals who do not typically take in information through sounds. Each and every day when you are in a safe space, when you are sitting down, turn off your visual senses and your kinesthetic senses and activate your hearing senses. Take into your body everything that you hear, however loud or soft; however abrasive or however sweet to the soul and heart. It does not matter what sounds you are hearing. Simply acknowledge them. Hear them with a fresh listening ear. Notice that the sounds come from many different places and sources. There are layers and layers on top of sounds once you begin to be attentive to them.

It is even more complicated however. We don't just hear sounds that are external to our body. There are also sounds that come from deep within our body. Our body actually makes noises all the time. Notice what noises your body is making internally. Simply hear and acknowledge those noises.

Finally, there is a sound that many people also hear; it is almost as though there is a voice outside of them talking - consoling them, even giving them advice. I have a very well-known songwriter friend who tells me that all of her songs are heard by her before she actually writes them. Where does that sound come from? Where does that music come from? She says she has no idea. It simply happens to be a gift that has been given to her from somewhere far, far away.

The invitation however doesn't have to do with these sounds that come from some place other than physical. Focus your attention on all physical sources of sounds whether they are external to you or internal in the sense of sounds that your body actually emits.

24

I now have a companion invitation that will fascinate all of you whether you happen to be kinesthetic, visual or auditory. As you are in bed and about ready to go to sleep, I invite you to cup both of your ears with your hands and listen to what you hear - to what sounds your body is making. Do it every night. Do it for at least a couple of minutes and if you are so motivated, keep your hands cupped for at least 10 minutes. Place your hands in a comfortable position so you don't have to hold them up – literally rest them on the pillow, cup and enjoy.

May you treasure each and every sound bite that you hear continuously throughout the week. Be sure that when you turn your full attention and focus to sounds that you are in a safe place, that you are seated and that you are not required to perform any particular duty or have any particular responsibility. It's important not to activate those new neural pathways if you are doing driving or operating heavy machinery, or doing anything that might result in injury.

May you delight in listening to sounds all week long. Some of you of course take in sounds as a matter of routine, so this challenge won't be new to you, but cupping your hands and listening to your body will.

Deeper Meaning Behind Noticing Sounds

What is then, the deeper meaning behind being mindful of hearing all of the sounds that surround you from outside your body as well as inside? What's the big deal here? We've been exposed to sounds long before we were even born.

Sound has a profound impact on our body. A new revolutionary approach for healing individuals is known as BioAcoustics. By listening to a 40 second sound track of my voice, BioAcoustics can identify what is out of balance in my body right now. This is done merely through the sound that I am now emitting from my body with my voice. Isn't that incredible?

The second phase of the therapy involves using sound to bring what is out of balance in my body back in. For example, if this analysis shows that I am deficient in Vitamin C, Vitamin C resonates at a very specific frequency. It is possible for me to get Vitamin C through the specific sound that is identified with the frequency that Vitamin C resonates at. Isn't that also incredible?

Everything in the body has a vibration. It is possible to diagnose and treat imbalances with sound. I believe this is one new medicine of the future. Medicines and supplements do the same thing. They vibrate at a specific frequency once they are ingested in our body. It is that vibration that winds up having the impact that it has. When a medicine has conflicting frequencies that are emitted, side effects result.

Did you notice over the last few days that certain sounds were grating to your body? There is no doubt about it. Some sounds create significant harm. Some sounds are dangerous. Be attentive to which sounds that were unpleasant or egregious to you. It may be the case that you are exposed to a sound that is not in your best and highest good. It may be in your best interest to eliminate that vibration or that sound, or move to a place where you are no longer exposed to that sound.

What music do you like to listen to? The music that you are attracted to has the tones that your body needs to hear. Listen to that music. It is truly and genuinely healing.

What is the business of cupping your ears all about? Now I know that is the mysterious and magical answer you have been waiting to hear (I say hear here rather than read because this week we are focusing on sound).

Our bodies naturally emit a vibration at a very, very low level. It sounds something like a refrigerator humming though even that is a derelict description. When you cupped your hands, you heard a sound humming or buzzing or vibrating inside your body. That, as it turns out, is precisely the sound that your body needs to receive to

27

come back into balance. By cupping your ears you are giving back to your body precisely the vibrations that it needs to have in order to come back into full balance and harmony. This is one means of returning to wellness.

Isn't that simple technique quite magical indeed? No diagnosis is necessary. No healthcare practitioners are required. This simple technique is available to you anytime of the day or night. It is simple. It takes a few minutes. It is easy to do. And best of all, it will always be free.

Your body is always emitting the frequencies that it needs to absorb. Listen to your body by cupping your ears. As you hear those vibrations, allow them to be returned to each and every cell of your body. In doing so, you are healing yourself. Now, if that's not cool I don't know what is.

Hum Hu

Do you find yourself thinking periodically that your body is unable to manufacture and produce dopamine naturally? Do you find that one of the thoughts that you believe to be true is that the cells your body needed to produce dopamine simply are dead and gone forever? I have gathered a compelling body of evidence which shows this thought to be blatantly false in most cases.

Person after person tell me a very similar story, though the details vary. Some have been guests on my radio show. Others have conveyed their experience during private conversations. The story, regardless of where or how it is conveyed, is consistent person after person after person.

Here is the template of the story I hear time and time again:

> *"When I was younger I loved to – [and here you have to fill the blank]. For example, I loved to play ping pong. When I developed symptoms of Parkinson's, I stopped playing ping pong. I felt like I did not have the motor skills to play anymore.*
>
> *One day I was inspired and I decided, "I think I will try and play a game of ping pong. After all, what do I have to lose?"*

> *Lo and behold, once that paddle and ball were in hand, all of my symptoms vanished. They no longer existed. You could not tell I had any neurological difficulties whatsoever. I could have been a professional player of ping pong and could beat literally anyone."*

My example centers on ping pong. I have heard story after story about many other activities including kickboxing, painting, woodwork, tennis, martial arts, boxing, skating, singing, knitting, sewing and others. Now if the body does not have the cells that are required to manufacture dopamine, I can assure you that none of those activities would be possible.

I also know that in doing meditations with groups, few symptoms surface after five or six minutes. At that point everyone is in a place of calmness and centeredness. If you meditate, doesn't this happen to you? Once you find that you calm your body down, you are no longer anxious. You are no longer tremoring.

The key then is to recognize that trauma and stress play leading roles in interrupting the neural pathways that are required for the body to manufacture dopamine. The body can do it, but when trauma obstructs the process, symptoms rear their ugly head.

How then can you sustain yourself in a place of serenity, in a place of centeredness, in a place of balance? How can you be present each and every moment, stress free? That of course is the purpose of these mindfulness challenges which will change habits that are no longer in our best and highest good.

One suggestion that I have for you (which came from one of my listeners who said it had helped him enormously) is to hum a word. What's the word you wonder? The word is HU. I'm not inventing this or making this up. Apparently this idea has roots that go back tens of thousands of years. People who were our great-great-great-great grandmothers and grandfathers were individuals who likely hummed this very same word. How does it actually sound?

When I listen to others humming HU, it sounds a lot like just the letter U. The challenge this week will be to hum the HU word several times a day or more frequently if you are so moved. Experiment with vocalizing this sound. You can usually shift pretty quickly into a place of calmness, a place of serenity and a place of balance. This is the place of serenity that activates the pathways that make dopamine.

Think about it. How often do you see a nervous cow? And, what do you hear cows say throughout the day? They know the value of humming HU. Certainly we can learn too!

Production of dopamine is interrupted when we are in a place of anxiety and stress. When trauma is present there is little chance you will be able to calm symptoms. However, when we are able to become centered, calm and serene - when stress no longer has a vice grip on our ego - we are able to activate all the processes in the body that are necessary to manufacture dopamine naturally.

Deeper Meaning Behind Humming HU

How has your experience with humming been coming along this week? How many times have you hummed every day? My experience is that the more often I Hum HU:

- *The better I feel.*
- *The calmer I feel.*
- *The happier I feel.*
- *The more I enjoy each and every moment.*
- *The more mindful I become of living in the present.*

What then is really happening when you and I hum the word HU? All of us carry a certain frequency. When we are moody or depressed, our frequency is very low. When we have negative thoughts like: "I'm going to never recover," a very low frequency resonates throughout our body.

Let me emphasize, I'm talking about a physical reality here. This is not a farfetched assertion. You can actually measure the frequency of the human energy field. It is a scientific phenomenon.

What we're really doing when we hum HU is that we, as it turns out, are raising our frequency higher and higher and higher, each time we hum. Isn't that cool! That's all you have to do.

We don't have to go to a therapist and talk for hours on end about all the pain and agony that we have suffered in our lifetime. We don't have to see our talk therapist every week for a decade. All we really need to do is to hum if we want to raise our frequency.

In the end, the highest frequency always wins out over the lower frequencies. When you resonate at the higher frequencies, the less likely it will be that the symptoms of Parkinson's have any prayer of rearing their ugly heads.

Continue to hum for the rest of the week and perhaps long thereafter. Remember - with each humming sequence you give yourself the gift of notching up the frequency of your energy field a notch or two. The more frequently you hum,

The higher your frequency,
The fewer your symptoms,
The greater your balance and serenity.

The possibility that your symptoms have any prayer of presenting themselves is smashed.

This has no religious roots whatsoever. Humming HU is not practiced by any religion. It is simply known to be a sound that raises the frequency of the human energy field. This is why this simple activity works.

I've heard back from a number of individuals who do this. They tell me you would not believe what this has done for them. It is simple to do. It is free. You can do it for yourself at any time of the day or night.

You will also know that the more you hum, the higher your frequency will resonate, the happier you will be, the more likely it is that all problems in your life will gently fade away into the sunset.

Hum away the rest of the week. Keep in mind you don't necessarily have to hum out loud, especially if you are with others or in a crowded space and are worried what people might be thinking in response to your humming. You can hum to yourself silently.

Consider adopting this as a regular mindful exercise that you can activate at any point in time – especially those moments and occasions when you feel yourself stressed and anxious. It is a gentle way to settle all of that down and move into a place where stress does not have a prayer of mucking up your neurological system.

Parkinsons Recovery Programs

Has your work on these exercises been stress free? Has it been helpful in reducing your symptoms? I certainly hope so! This is the primary reason I developed the mindfulness exercises in the first place.

If you struggled with pacing out these mindfulness exercises so as not to induce more stress, there are several Parkinsons Recovery programs that might help expedite your recovery. My Parkinsons Recovery Mindfulness Program sends the mindfulness exercises in an email to you each and every week. The initial exercise is sent to your email address on day one of the week and the deeper implications are sent four days later. The Parkinsons Recovery Mindfulness Program takes one full year to complete as each exercise is introduced one week at a time. For more information visit:

www.stress.parkinsonsrecovery.com

Parkinsons Recovery Memberships involve a variety of support websites that are essential to recovery. A difference mindfulness exercise is posted each week. For more information on Parkinsons Recovery memberships visit:

www.parkinsonsrecovery.org

Of course, the approach that works for many people is to purchase a single volume of the Parkinsons Recovery Mindfulness program at a time as you have already done! See the introduction for a listing of all nine Parkinsons Recovery Mindfulness volumes.

Thank you for Your Support

On behalf of the thousands of followers of Parkinsons Recovery, I want to thank you for your purchase of this booklet. One hundred percent (100%) of the profits purchases of my books and programs help subsidize the many free services I offer through Parkinsons Recovery -

www.parkinsonsrecovery.com

For information about other products, services and programs visit -

www.parkinsonsrecovery.me